C000149362

A Survivor's Guide To
Healthy Living

Chris McLaughlin

Medical Editor
Dr Tony Smith

Published by Family Doctor Publications
in association with the British Medical Association

Medical Editor: Dr Tony Smith
Front Cover Illustration: Colette Blanchard
Illustrators: Ilona Tate, Alex Harwood
Design: Neil Deacon
Printing: Cambus Litho, Scotland, using acid-free paper

ISBN: 1 898205 19 1

Contents

BRITISH MEDICAL ASSOCIATION

Survival of the fittest

Those of us alive in Britain now can expect to live longer than any previous generation – with the average life expectancy being about 75 for men and 80 for women. Like all averages, however, these figures conceal as much as they reveal. For one thing, half the population will not in fact make it to these ages, and around a quarter of us will die before the age of 65. The odds of surviving into the seventies and beyond are not the same for men and women, with many more men dying prematurely. As we'll see in the next chapter, many of those who don't live into old age die of illnesses which might have been prevented.

Prevention is mostly a matter of lifestyle. The importance of how we live in determining how and when we die is becoming ever clearer. For example, non-smokers who eat a healthy diet, take reasonable amounts of exercise and drink only moderately are less likely to succumb to a variety of potentially lethal conditions than those who don't follow such guidelines. Of course, this is not to say that a person who suffers a fatal illness at a relatively early age has only him- or herself to blame, but it does mean that you can improve your chances of avoiding many such illnesses by making changes to the way you live.

It's not only fatal illnesses that may be linked to lifestyle. Many of the disabling ill-

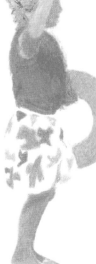

nesses which could otherwise spoil the quality of life in your later years may be preventable or at least reduced in severity by looking after your health and taking an informed interest in how your condition is treated.

The aim of this book is not to tell you how to live your life or make you feel guilt-ridden about any 'bad' habits, still less to frighten or depress you. The real message is a much more positive one: by giving you the facts about the links between health and lifestyle, we hope to dispel any fears and confusion resulting from the frequent scare stories in the media so you can

make an informed choice about the way you want to live.

Of course, there's not much attraction in the prospect of living longer if it means giving up everything that makes life worthwhile. 'Healthy living' isn't all about self-denial, but about the positive gains you can make in terms of feeling good for as long as possible.

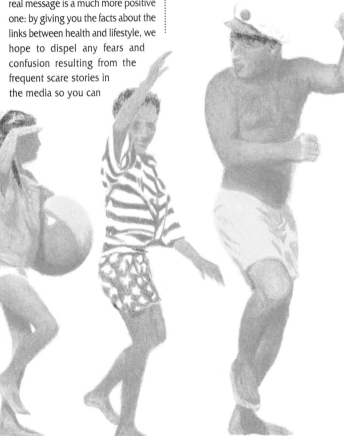

Identifying the killers

While there's no avoiding the fact that we all have to die some time, by following the advice in this you can improve your chances of avoiding death before you've lived out your normal lifespan. Each year, 60,000 men and 37,000 women die before the age of 65, and it is these deaths of people 'too young to die' which are our main target.

As we've seen, a woman can expect to outlive a man on average, and the gap doesn't seem to be closing.

Under 30s

The reasons why people die prematurely vary greatly depending on their ages. In a typical year in England and Wales, around 4,400 men and 1,800 women die before the age of 30. Although such deaths may have been commonplace in the past, today we see them as unnatural, and rightly so. Some are due to genuine accidents – such as being struck by lightning or hit by a tree blown over in a gale – but most are at least partly preventable. Although a few young adults die

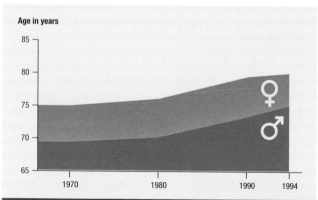

Male (♂) and female (♀) life expectancy

from conditions such as cystic fibrosis (a disease due to an inborn lack of certain enzymes or body chemicals in the lungs), most deaths are due to injury or poisoning rather than illness.

In fact, the most significant cause of death is road accidents, which kill around 4,000 people every year (around 1,400 of them, mostly males, aged under 30). These account for most of the deaths listed as 'violent', and explain why the figures are higher for men than for women. It is possible to reduce these numbers, and accident prevention is discussed in greater detail in the next chapter. Suicide is another important cause of death in this age group, but coroners' juries are reluctant to bring in a verdict of suicide unless the evidence is overwhelming. The truth is that most deaths from poisoning are actually suicides, but these are far from easy to prevent. Telephone counselling by groups such as the Samaritans may be helpful, but improvements are also needed in the community care of people with long-term illnesses such as schizophrenia.

Between 31 and 50

In this age group, accidents are still a major cause of death, but some people also die from heart disease or strokes, as well as a few from infections.

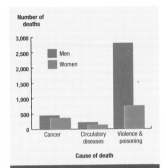

Causes of death among those aged 15–30

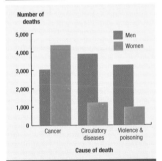

Causes of death among those aged 30–50

Some people in this age group die from illnesses which have a genetic component: for example, women with breast cancer usually suffer from the rare, inherited, familial kind, while victims of heart disease have usually inherited a biochemical defect that pushes the blood cholesterol to very high levels. However, the fact that you have inherited a high risk of developing a particular disease does not mean that you will necessarily do so. You can find out

8

more about prevention and screening in the next chapter.

From 50 to 65

When we look at the causes of death in people in this age group, it is clear that accidents are now a much smaller percentage, while heart attacks, strokes and cancers have become more common. The death rate for men in this age group is so much higher than women's largely because men are more vulnerable to heart attacks. It is at this time in their lives that people are likely to succumb to diseases that are often partly related to smoking.

Family factors

In most cases where people die from disease before the age of 65, there will usually be inherited and lifestyle factors involved. To see how these might affect you personally, look at your close

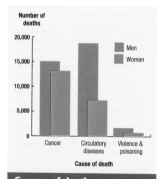

Causes of death among those aged 50–65

relatives. If most of them have lived until 80 or longer, you have little to worry about.

On the other hand, if one or more of your blood relatives has died from disease before they reached 65, you should find out the exact cause. 'Cancer', for example, is not enough – you need to know where it started. Then ask your doctor for advice. Often there will be screening tests available: for instance, if strokes have affected your family, your blood pressure will need to be checked.

Beyond 65

Beyond the age of 65, illness becomes more common, but it still isn't inevitable. You could be one of the many people whose health remains good and who suffer little decline in general fitness until they're gone 80. A few people even manage to compete in marathons at this age! Once again, looking at your family should be your main guide to any health hazards which may lie ahead for you too: were your parents, aunts and uncles overweight? Did they smoke themselves to death? Did they have cancer, and if so, what kind? This may all sound rather morbid, but it doesn't mean you must become obsessed with death. The aim is to identify any possible risk areas for yourself which you can then – with medical help – steer clear of.

Staying alive

None of us will live for ever, but it makes sense to do everything within reason to avoid dying before our time. Perhaps even more important is quality of life. Many chronic conditions may not kill you, but they make it difficult if not impossible to enjoy life to the full.

Avoiding accidents

As we've seen, younger people face a very real risk of suffering death or serious injury as the result of an accident. Some will always be completely unpredictable and perhaps unavoidable, but many could definitely have been prevented with a little forethought. Interestingly, research suggests that while cars are becoming safer, and legislation such as compulsory wearing of seat belts ought to reduce the numbers of serious injuries and deaths, this is not happening in practice. It may be that some drivers are opting for more powerful cars, driving faster and taking greater risks because the safety improvements make them overconfident. This has severe consequences for pedestrians and cyclists in particular – and the numbers of them injured and killed are rising. Pedestrians should dress to ensure they can be seen at night, while cyclists should make sure their lights work, wear something fluorescent and a crash helmet.

9

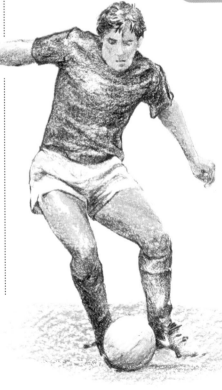

Play safe

While there's no doubt that taking part in sport brings health bonuses, it can be hazardous too if you're not careful. It's been estimated that there are around 19 million injuries caused by sporting activities every year, and although deaths are relatively rare, they do happen. Around half of all injuries are suffered by young men between 16 and 25, and although rugby is the riskiest game, more people actually get hurt during soccer matches, partly because more people play this kind of football.

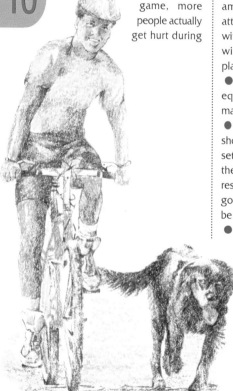

Genuine accidents are sometimes unavoidable, but you can improve your chances of coming through unscathed with a few simple precautions:

● Get fit before you join in anything which is very physically demanding.

● Competitive sport has a higher injury rate, especially among keen amateurs who take a cavalier attitude to safety. Avoid playing with those who think rules are for wimps, and who delight in playing dirty.

● Make sure you have the correct equipment for your sport and maintain it properly if necessary.

● Hill walkers and climbers should check the weather before setting out, make sure they have the right gear, and always tell a responsible person where they're going and when they expect to be back.

● Don't be over-confident: it's foolhardy to go climbing, sailing or caving, for example, unless you really know what you're doing, and even then the hazards can be very real.

● Never mix alcohol and any kind of watersports.

● Stick rigidly to safety rules and don't take chances.

10

Reducing the risk

● Alcohol is the commonest factor in all accidents, whether on the road, at home or at work. You need to be extra careful when you've been drinking, and avoid situations where you could be at risk, such as crossing a busy road. Of course, you should never drink and drive or travel with anyone who does.

● Falls are responsible for many of the injuries and some deaths, especially among the very young and the elderly. Check out potential hazards, such as loose carpets and slippery floors, broken stair-rails, steep steps and the like, to make your environment at home and at work as safe as possible.

● Older people in particular should make sure they have powerful lightbulbs on stairways and in halls or corridors to reduce the chances of falling over something unseen. A recent survey showed that over half a million people were injured in 1993 as a result of either falling down stairs or colliding with furniture – and bad lighting obviously must have played a part in many cases.

● The same survey revealed 200,000 cases of injury to people carrying out DIY jobs in the home. Apparently Sunday evening is the riskiest time when there is a rush to get the job finished – so be warned!

● Make sure you have smoke alarms and fire extinguishers fitted in your home, and check them regularly according to the makers' instructions.

● Accidental poisoning mostly affects children – whether it be from swallowing cleaning fluids, for example, or helping themselves from the medicine cabinet. The answer here is to ensure that anything potentially dangerous is locked away so there is no chance of a child getting at things he shouldn't while your back is turned.

● It's easy to be complacent and assume that accidents only happen to other people. The best way to reduce the risk is to be aware that it could be your turn next unless you develop your safety consciousness and do what you can to stay out of potentially dangerous situations.

11

Hazards at work

Unfortunately, some jobs carry an inbuilt element of risk, and there usually isn't a lot the individual can do about the fact. Even changing your job isn't a realistic option for many people these days.

Companies operating in industries where the dangers are greatest, such as offshore oil and gas rigs, construction and deep sea fishing, are well aware of the hazards, and most take rigorous precautions to protect their employees as far as possible. Workers in these environments often face strict controls – such as the banning of alcohol on offshore rigs – and have extensive safety training. Beyond this, it is up to the individual to take care of himself as far as possible – making proper use of safety equipment and protective clothing, for example, and making sure machinery guards and other safety devices are in place and properly maintained. It can be tempting to cut corners to save time or make a task easier, but the price can be high if you're unlucky.

You may be concerned if you know that you come into contact at work with known cancer-causing agents (carcinogens) – such as asbestos, benzene, certain cutting oils and chemicals, for example. Your employer is legally obliged to tell you that you are working with any toxic substances and is responsible for ensuring that you are as well protected from them as possible. You should raise any worries you have about safety with your employer or union representative if you have one, and there should be someone appointed as safety representative. You can get outside advice if necessary from your local Employment Medical Adviser; the number will be in the phone book under the Health and Safety Executive.

Avoiding illness
Heart disease

As we saw in the previous chapter, diseases of the circulatory system (such as heart disease and strokes) are responsible for many premature deaths. Up to around 50, men are much more susceptible to coronary heart disease than women. However, a woman faces an increasing risk after the menopause because she is no longer protected by the female hormone oestrogen unless she is taking hormone replacement therapy (HRT).

While there is a lot you can do to reduce your chances of developing heart disease, some of the factors involved are more or less outside your control. For example, you can't change your sex nor can you avoid getting older – which means that you can't prevent your cardiovascular system becoming less efficient as the years pass. You may also be at increased risk if several close family members have suffered a heart attack, although it is difficult to tell whether it is some aspect of your genetic inheritance or the shared family lifestyle that is helping to load the dice against you. For example, you may have a tendency to high blood pressure or to raised levels of cholesterol which is partly genetically determined. On the other hand, you may also have followed the example of family members by eating an 'unhealthy' diet (and possibly putting on a lot of weight), smoking and taking virtually no exercise.

A recent government survey found that almost nine out of ten adults have one or more of the main risk factors for heart disease which could be reduced by changes in lifestyle. The major culprits are smoking, high blood pressure and raised cholesterol, but the wrong kind of diet, obesity, inactivity and certain other illnesses such as diabetes can all add to the risk, as can stress. In particular, the survey revealed that 13 per cent of men and 16 per cent of women were obese, with many more overweight to a less dramatic extent. (For more on this, see pages 51–2.) Only 10 per cent of those interviewed for the survey were free from four important avoidable heart disease risk factors: smoking, raised cholesterol, raised blood pressure and lack of exercise.

> **A recent government survey found that almost nine out of ten adults have one or more of the main risk factors for heart disease**

If your family is known to be particularly prone to heart disease, and especially if you have one or more of the other risk factors, your doctor may well suggest you have some tests. The most common tests are regular blood pressure checks, plus blood tests to measure your cholesterol level. You can be given treatment and other lifestyle advice to help bring both down towards normal levels if necessary.

Other changes are in your hands. The one that will make the most dramatic difference in terms of risk reduction is for a smoker to give up. Everyone who smokes can't help but be aware of the damage the weed does to their health, and many would love to stop if only they could. Once you have decided that you do want to stop, there's no shortage of help on offer.

13

Apart from having any tests and/or treatment your doctor thinks necessary, you can best reduce your chances of having a heart attack by paying attention to your diet and by getting more exercise. You'll find detailed guidelines on how to do this in the next chapter.

Stroke

Much the same applies to strokes – which is when a clot or bleeding affecting one of the blood vessels in your brain causes damage to the surrounding tissue. Usually this is the result of damage to your blood vessels which has been happening over the course of many years. In more than half the cases of stroke, the factor mainly responsible for the damage is raised blood pressure, but smoking, being overweight, excessive drinking and a high salt intake can also play their part. Regular blood pressure checks will pick up any rise in the early stages before too much harm has been done. Your doctor will decide what treatment, if any, is necessary, but will also expect you to do your bit by adopting as healthy a lifestyle as you can.

Cancer

The first thing to understand is that cancer is not one single disease but many. What all forms of the disease have in common is that cell division runs out of control and the abnormal cells cluster together to form a tumour. This change in cell behaviour can be triggered by a variety of factors, but some experts estimate that around 80 per cent of cancers may be preventable by adopting a healthy lifestyle and improving the environment.

> **Smokers who get through a packet a day are 20 times more likely to get lung cancer than non-smokers**

Some types of cancer can run in families, although most sufferers will not have had an affected relative. If two or more members of your immediate family (that is, your blood relatives) have died of the same type of cancer before the age of 65, ask your doctor to refer you to a cancer specialist for checks. It is important to be sure exactly what their illness was – 'cancer' by itself is too vague. The cancers which may run in families (although usually they don't) include breast, ovary and bowel.

Smoking: this is undoubtedly the biggest cause of avoidable cancer – around a third of cancer deaths are smoking-related, including some of the commonest forms such as cancers of the lung, pancreas, oesophagus, bladder

14

and cervix. Smokers who get through a packet a day are 20 times more likely to get lung cancer than non-smokers, and nearly 44,000 people die of it every year. There are said to be around 4,000 different chemicals in tobacco smoke, and while no one knows what each one does, they can affect every part of your body. Two chemicals in particular – nicotine and carbon monoxide – are thought to be responsible for much of the damage. Some of the effects are obvious, such as the destruction of the air sacs in the lungs, for example, while others are more subtle and can involve damaging changes at the cell level, triggering the production of a tumour. For advice on giving up see pages 47–8.

Alcohol: people who both smoke and drink a lot are more likely to suffer from throat cancer, and excessive drinking is also related to the development of cancers in the mouth, oesophagus and liver. This doesn't mean that drinking alcohol is bad for you as such; in fact, there is some evidence that people who drink one or two units of alcohol (see page 16 for explanation of units) have a lower risk of heart disease than those who drink no alcohol at all or those who drink more than two units. In other words, the secret of safe drinking is

15

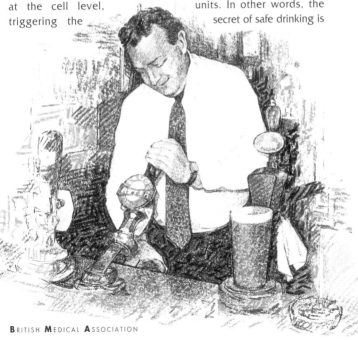

moderation. Men should stick to 28 units or less of alcohol, while for women the limit is 21 units per week. Try to steer clear of alcohol completely for one or two days every week, and spread out your allowance over several days rather than downing it all in one epic drinking session.

Sex: experts believe that there may be a link between sexually transmitted viruses and certain kinds of cancer – particularly those of the anus and the cervix. In general, the more sexual relationships you (or your regular partner) have, the greater the possible risk. There is also a suggestion that's a woman's chances of developing cervical cancer may be higher if she started having sex at a relatively young age. Of course, you can't undo the past, but regular smear tests will make sure that any early signs of developing cancer will be picked up at an early stage when they can be effectively treated. Using barrier methods of contraception such as the male or female condom or the diaphragm can also offer a woman some protection.

At work: your job may bring you into contact with substances that have the potential to cause cancer in the long term and it is vital to take all possible precautions to protect yourself. For more on this, see page 12.

Sun: skin cancer is the second most common kind of cancer and is largely caused by exposure to ultraviolet (UV) light from the sun. Cases have risen in line with the

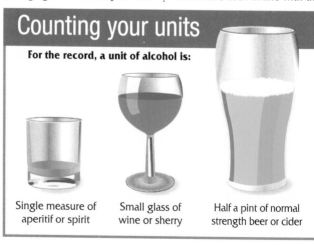

Counting your units

For the record, a unit of alcohol is:

Single measure of aperitif or spirit

Small glass of wine or sherry

Half a pint of normal strength beer or cider

HIV and AIDS

No one knows how many people in this country may be carrying HIV (or human immunodeficiency virus). Although the majority of people already diagnosed acquired the infection through homosexual sex or using contaminated equipment for injecting drugs, there are many more who have become infected through heterosexual sex and don't yet know it. When they do find out – either because they have a test or develop signs of the acquired immune deficiency syndrome (AIDS) – most will probably have no idea from whom they got it. A person who is HIV positive may feel and look perfectly well for many years, even though they are capable of passing the infection to other people.

The virus can be passed on from an infected person during unprotected sex – in other words, when the man is not wearing a condom. It can be transmitted from man to woman or vice versa or from one man to another during anal intercourse. The risk is thought to be less during oral sex, but it can happen. Unless you know for certain that your partner is not HIV positive, it is risky to have sex unless the man is wearing a condom – which should be one of those carrying the British Standards Institution symbol as a guarantee of quality.

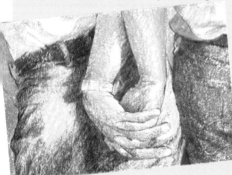

The AIDS virus is carried in body fluids, which include blood, and this is why there may be some risk in certain countries from medical treatment involving the use of syringes, needles and blood transfusions. If you're planning a journey to a country where the standards of medical care may be dubious, it's a good idea to consult your GP or MASTA (see page 20) about whether you should take your own travel medical kit. These are available from MASTA and many pharmacies.

increasing popularity of sunshine holidays abroad. The only way to minimise your risk is to remain well covered when out in the sun, even in this country, and to avoid sunbathing altogether. Regular application of sunscreen with an appropriate SPF (sun protection factor) is an extra precaution, not an alternative. The level of protection you need will depend on your skin type and the intensity of the sun that you're going to be exposed to. You'll find guidelines on the packaging, or you can ask the pharmacist for help. If you're not sure which one to choose, remember that UV rays can penetrate cloud, and can also be reflected from your surroundings even when you're in the shade.

Diet: researchers are still studying the possible links, but some estimates suggest that as many as 35 per cent of cancers may be food-related. In particular, there is thought to be a connection with cancers of the oesophagus, breast, stomach, bowel and prostate. Being obese may in itself increase your

18

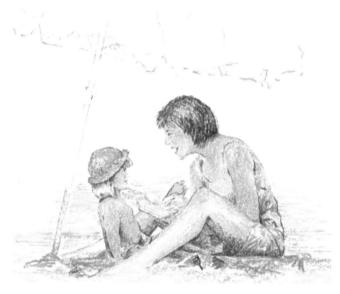

Skin cancer – what to look for

Although still the rarest type of skin cancer, malignant melanoma has one of the fastest rates of increase of all cancers and is lethal if allowed to spread. It develops rapidly, with changes taking weeks or months rather than years.

The risk is greatest for those who have:
- a lot of moles (say more than 50), especially if they look irregular in shape or colour
- red or fair hair, fair skin and freckles, blue eyes
- trouble getting a really 'good' tan but burn easily
- two or more relatives who have suffered from this type of skin cancer.

Any brown mark on the skin which matches up with any of the points listed below should be seen straight away by a doctor.
- A mole or brown or black spot which grows, especially in an adult of 35 or more. A growing mole means one which is extending across more of the skin surface – becoming more rounded or raised up is not significant. Any mark that is bigger than the blunt end of a pencil should be checked out.
- A mark which has an irregularly shaped outline or surface, unlike a mole which is likely to be symmetrical.
- Variation in colour – a mark that is a mixture of brown and black, or possibly red or with a bluish-white tinge. A mole that suddenly develops a red or pink tinge should be investigated.

The other two types of skin cancer are:
- Basal cell carcinoma: this is the most common but least dangerous type; it is sometimes referred to as rodent ulcer because, if untreated, it causes a deep cavity as if the skin had been eaten by a rat. Unlike all other forms of cancer, it never spreads to other parts of the body, but, if left untreated, it can become very large and so cause bad disfigurement.
- Squamous cell carcinoma: although less common, this form of cancer is more dangerous in that it can spread if not treated and can ultimately be fatal. Red, thick, scaling patches, usually on the face or hands, are the first signs, and if left they may evolve into raised, red growths with a warty surface.

19

vulnerability to some cancers, so it really is worth making the effort to lose weight if necessary. Even if your weight is within the normal range, you should follow the healthy eating guidelines in the next chapter. The most valuable change you can make is to eat more fresh fruit and vegetables – ideally five portions a day – and cut down on the amount of fat you consume. Aim to have no more than one-third of your total daily calorie intake in the form of fat.

Infections

Although there are occasional deaths from infectious diseases caught in this country, such as Legionnaires' disease, meningitis and even salmonella in the elderly, there has also been an alarming rise in the number of people coming back from foreign holidays with potentially serious illnesses.

Malaria is probably the most serious problem: over 2,000 people are infected every year and more than half of them have the potentially fatal form known as falciparum malaria caused by *Plasmodium falciparum*. Most of them have been to Africa, with destinations such as the Gambia,

Kenya, Tanzania and Zimbabwe carrying particularly high risks.

Anyone who is planning to travel outside Europe, North America or Australia should consult their GP or a specialist travel clinic such as those run by British Airways or the Medical Advisory Service for Travellers Abroad (MASTA) (tel: 0171 631 4408) for advice on the necessary precautions. In some areas, you may also need immunisation against other unpleasant illnesses which can lurk in exotic destinations, so you'll need to get organised several weeks before departure to make sure you're fully protected. Even the most stringent precautions are not guaranteed to stop you getting malaria, unfortunately, so don't hesitate to go to your doctor if you feel ill on your return, and remind him or her about where you've just been. Stomach upsets and diarrhoea are often a minor nuisance on long-haul trips, and most cases of 'Delhi belly' or 'Montezuma's revenge' are not serious. However, you should consult your doctor if your symptoms don't go away or start after you come back in case you have picked up something which needs treatment.

In good
health

Sadly, many people who do beat the odds by living on into their seventies and eighties also develop disabling conditions which rob them of the chance to really enjoy those extra years. Some of them will have had their illnesses for years and find that they get worse with age; others may develop conditions which are ultimately fatal but which restrict their activities and ability to enjoy life to the full well before that.

In 1993, 63 per cent of men and 66 per cent of women aged over 65 said they suffered from poor health. The main causes included mental illness, disorders of the heart and circulation, and problems with muscles and joints.

While it may be impossible to avoid such illnesses entirely, there is often a lot you can do to keep on top of them by learning as much as you can and doing all you can to control the condition.

Arthritis

Stiff, swollen and painful joints are the main symptom of the two best-known types of arthritis – osteo-arthritis and rheumatoid arthritis.

Osteoarthritis, which is often called the 'wear and tear' disease, usually affects older people, although it can begin at a relatively early age, and professional sports people often suffer if their joints have been damaged through injury. Rheumatoid arthritis usually begins in the 30s or 40s, and like osteoarthritis, it tends to run in families. Drugs are available to reduce inflammation and to ease the pain, and surgery may also be an option when joints are badly damaged.

While there is nothing much you can do to stop yourself developing arthritis, learning about your condition and your treatment can make a difference. It is important to keep your muscles in good working order, but exercise should be properly geared to your state of health, and a physiotherapist is the best person to advise you. Keeping your weight down to within the normal range will also help by reducing the strain on your joints. With rheumatoid arthritis in particular, the balance between the benefits of some drug treatments and the possible side effects can be a delicate one, so the greater your knowledge and understanding, the more you can contribute to the successful management of your condition.

There have been some reports linking special diets with improvements in symptoms, but there is as yet no real evidence that this works for the majority of people with arthritis. In any case, you shouldn't make any dramatic changes to your diet without expert advice.

Depression

Depression is an illness which can strike anyone at any time, yet many sufferers don't seek help because they don't realise that treatment is available. Sadly, many people also feel embarrassed to admit they are depressed, as though it were somehow their own fault, and feel they should just 'pull themselves together'. In fact, there is no reason to suffer in silence. While a bout of depression may eventually go away on its own, it's far better to seek help from your GP at an early stage as there are various kinds of treatment which can help you recover more quickly.

Depression has some features in common with sadness or a passing low mood, but there are other symptoms which set it apart. Depression and anxiety are the most common features, but sufferers are likely to experience other difficulties too.

No one knows what triggers depressive illness. In some people, it may begin after some specific event in their lives, but others may find that it just creeps up on them without warning.

Symptoms of depression

- tiredness ● headache and palpitations
- inability to get pleasure from activities you previously enjoyed
- disturbed sleep, difficulty in getting to sleep or waking early with black thoughts
- feeling irritable and short-tempered
- loss of interest in sex
- finding it difficult to concentrate, even on a TV programme, not to mention everyday tasks
- loss of appetite or, less commonly, over-eating
- suicidal thoughts

All of these symptoms are caused directly or indirectly by changes in the levels of chemicals in some areas of your brain. As you begin to recover, either spontaneously or with treatment, the levels begin returning to normal.

23

Treatment

The main thing you have to remember is that, however negative and hopeless you feel at the moment, depression does get better. Treatment including drugs and counselling can help most people to recover more quickly.

● Antidepressant drugs work by treating the chemical imbalance in your brain, and returning it towards the normal. You cannot become addicted to them, but if you have had several episodes of depression,

you may be prescribed long-term treatment.

● Counselling involves talking about how you feel. Some people find talking to family and friends a great help, but it is often easier to be honest with an outsider such as a trained counsellor. Your GP, practice nurse or counsellor, a clinical psychologist or a psychiatrist can all provide this kind of therapy.

Helping yourself

While you can't just snap out of

24

depression, there are some positive steps you can take.

● Try to take each day as it comes

● Try to get some exercise every day, even if it's only a walk, however tired and lethargic you feel. The less you do, the more exhausted you will feel.

● Try not to take on more than you can realistically do. Concentrate on what you feel are the priorities and take a pride in what you achieve, even if it is less than you used to be able to do.

● Don't get too despondent if you have the odd really bad day. Try to look at the general trend – is this week or month better than the last one?

● If you ever feel suicidal, tell someone, such as your doctor, counsellor or the Samaritans.

Chest disease

Some people are born with a tendency to develop chronic lung diseases such as bronchitis or emphysema, but the main causes are smoking and certain kinds of air pollution, especially sulphur dioxide. In both cases, breathlessness is a major problem, and people with bronchitis will also suffer from excess mucus in the lungs and coughing. People with either of these conditions (which often go together in practice) may get frequent infections, and are often given antibiotics to keep ready so that they can begin treatment as soon as the first symptoms appear.

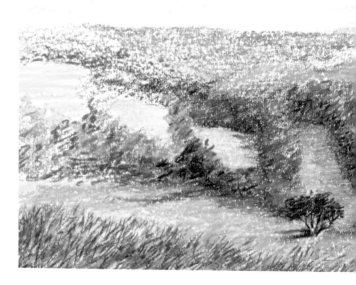

Earlier this century, sufferers from chronic chest diseases like these were sent to recuperate in healthier climates such as North Africa or the south of France, but unfortunately the NHS doesn't run to that these days. The principle still holds, however, and it is important to do what you can to ensure that you spend as much time as possible in a clean, smoke- and pollution-free environment. It goes without saying that you shouldn't smoke yourself, and it is a big help if family and visitors can be persuaded to abstain in your home too. You may well have physiotherapy to help clear your lungs, and your physio will advise you to keep as fit as you can and take as much exercise as you can manage. Keep an eye on the weather forecast, which these days include predictions of air quality. Certain weather conditions make high concentrations of atmospheric pollutants more likely, and it is wise to stay indoors on days when conditions are bad.

Asthma, as any sufferer knows, can come and go without any obvious explanation. Some people who suffer badly as children find it disappears altogether as they grow up, but it can also strike for the first time in the middle years or get worse as you get older.

Attacks can be triggered by a whole range of different factors, and it is important for an asthma sufferer to get to know what affects them personally. Viruses such as colds are a problem for many people, but

25

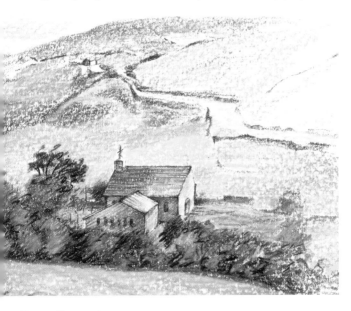

others react to allergens such as dust or animal fur, drugs, stress or atmospheric pollution, for example. Obviously it makes sense to avoid your own particular triggers as far as possible, but even more important is to understand your treatment and how to get maximum benefit from it. When you're feeling well, it's easy to become casual about using your preventer inhaler every day, but it is important not to neglect this as it does help to keep the lung inflammation at bay. You should also discuss with your doctor how to spot the early signs of an acute attack, and have an agreed plan of action to follow if one does happen. Like people with emphysema or bronchitis, you should keep an eye on weather forecasts and try to stay in when pollution levels are high (see page 56).

Diabetes

Diabetes is caused when a person's natural supply of insulin, a hormone produced by the pancreas, either fails completely or stops working efficiently. The result is that levels of glucose in the bloodstream are not kept under proper control, and fluctuate dramatically if the problem is not recognised and dealt with. One form of the condition (insulin-dependent diabetes (IDD) or type I) starts when the person is quite young, often around 12 or so; the other (non-insulin dependent diabetes or type II) normally strikes in middle age or

later. Although there is a tendency for diabetes, especially NIDDM (or type II), to run in families, lifestyle can also make it more likely that a susceptible person will develop NIDDM later on. Being overweight, eating too many fatty and sugary foods and lack of exercise are the main factors, so this is yet another good reason for following the healthy living guidelines in the next chapter.

The picture most of us have of diabetes is of the person having to give himself or herself daily injections of insulin to avoid going into a coma. In fact, it is usually only people with IDDM who have to do this, and diabetic comas are pretty rare. The majority of people with diabetes have the non-insulin-dependent kind and control it through healthy eating and often tablets as well. In either case, the aim of treatment is to keep levels of glucose in the bloodstream as close to normal as possible, to make up for the fact that the natural supply of insulin is not working as it should. Getting this balance right is very much an individual matter, and people with diabetes are encouraged to learn as much as they can about what works best for them personally.

When diabetes is undiagnosed or poorly controlled, complications can develop which may affect the eyes, the kidney, the heart and the nervous system, so regular check-ups and insight into the management of the condition are vital to minimise the risks.

26

First steps to a healthier lifestyle

L et's be clear about one thing: opting for a healthy lifestyle doesn't mean giving up everything you enjoy for the sake of better health. While it will mean changes, they can be made gradually and relatively painlessly if you set about it in the right way. And the good news is that, within weeks, you'll already be feeling and looking so much better, you won't want to go back to your old ways.

As we've seen, a healthy lifestyle will help protect you against various diseases, but in reality that knowledge isn't always a big enough incentive to change the way you live.

You can always kid yourself that it won't happen to you anyway, even when you know in your heart that's unlikely to be true. So if you need more of a kick start, concentrate instead on what you'll gain in the short term:

● You may lose weight once you start eating a healthy diet, even though it's not specifically intended for would-be slimmers

● You'll have far more energy (both physical and mental) than before

● You'll sleep better than you used to and wake feeling refreshed

● You'll feel calmer and better able to cope with everyday stress

● You'll feel much fitter –

running for a bus or climbing stairs won't leave you breathless
● You'll suffer fewer minor aches and pains – like backache and PMS (pre-menstrual syndrome)
● Your hair and skin will look better and your eyes clearer.

Once you have made up your mind to make some changes in the way you live, there are three main aspects to think about:
● Changing to a healthier diet
● Getting more exercise
● Learning to live with stress
And for smokers, there's another priority which should head your list – giving up can do more for your health (and your survival prospects) than   just about anything else. More on this on pages 48–9.

28

What's on the menu?

If your favourite meal happens to be a cheeseburger and fries, or you can't imagine life without chocolate, don't despair. While experts agree that neither are particularly good for you, they also agree that there's no such thing as a bad food, only a bad diet. In other words, you can safely indulge yourself every so often provided you eat a healthy diet the rest of the time. And healthy doesn't mean dull or tasteless. Experts believe that one of the healthiest patterns of eating is that enjoyed by people who live

around the shores of the Mediterranean. All the latest research points to the fact that in that part of the world, people have traditionally gone for the

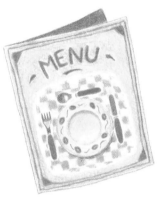

kinds of foods which offer the greatest health benefits, while at the same time eating little or none of those (such as animal fats) which may not be so good for us.

If you've ever been on holiday in southern Europe or North Africa, you know that the local people eat lots of fish, vegetables, fruit and salad, accompanied by rice and pasta, pulses and nuts, dressed with olive oil and fresh herbs, and very little red meat and dairy products. That means they get masses of vitamins and anti-oxidants, plenty of fish and natural fibre, while being sparing with sugar and the animal fats found in red meat and dairy foods. There is increasing evidence that this kind of diet can help to protect you

Starchy foods

These include bread, potatoes, pasta, rice, breakfast cereals and noodles. Think of this type of food as the base around which you plan a meal rather than as an accompaniment – say baked potatoes filled with cottage cheese or tuna, served with a salad, instead of roast meat with roast potatoes and vegetables. Contrary to what many people believe, starchy foods are not particularly fattening on their own, but of course adding lashings of butter or rich sauces will soon pile on the calories. As well as being filling, starchy foods are rich in minerals and other nutrients, and are also a good supply of fibre – an essential ingredient in your healthy eating plan.

Fibre (or roughage as it used to be called) is made up of the cell walls of plant foods – grains, leaves, roots and so on. Your system can't actually digest it, so it passes straight through you, picking up water and residues from the food you've eaten. It's been known for years that in societies where high-fibre diets are the norm, people suffer fewer diseases of the digestive system (including cancer) – and constipation is virtually unheard of! In addition, soluble fibre which is found in fruit, vegetables and oats, helps lower the levels of cholesterol in the bloodstream. Remember though that increasing your intake dramatically overnight can leave you feeling full of wind, so go slowly at first if you're not used to it.

29

from developing heart disease and certain kinds of cancer.

The variations of this kind of cooking are endless with something to please everyone. What's more, it's really very easy to apply the principles that make the Mediterranean diet a healthy one to your own everyday eating plan. It doesn't have to cost a fortune, especially if you choose food that's in season, and it doesn't mean spending hours in the kitchen either. Remember that you don't have to bring in all the changes overnight. If you prefer to take it slowly, especially if you are preparing meals for other members of the family who like what they're used to eating, you can adapt the menu gradually. To make meal-planning easier, aim to include some foods from each of the four main groups every day:

- Starchy foods
- Meat and alternatives
- Dairy products
- Vegetables (including salad and fruit).

Dairy products

Milk, cheese, fromage frais and yogurt. Supermarket shelves are crammed with reduced or low-fat versions of most dairy foods. Substituting semi-skimmed or skimmed milk for full cream and using a low-fat spread instead of butter most if not all of the time will make an enormous difference to your fat intake without making your tastebuds suffer noticeably. Keep cream and thick creamy yogurts for special occasions.

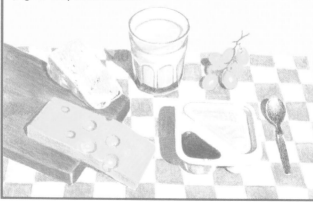

30

Meat and alternatives

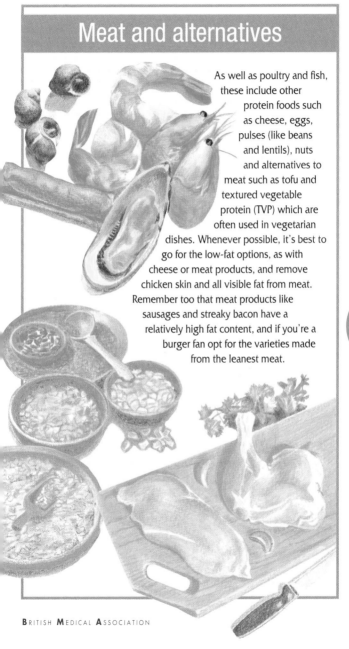

As well as poultry and fish, these include other protein foods such as cheese, eggs, pulses (like beans and lentils), nuts and alternatives to meat such as tofu and textured vegetable protein (TVP) which are often used in vegetarian dishes. Whenever possible, it's best to go for the low-fat options, as with cheese or meat products, and remove chicken skin and all visible fat from meat. Remember too that meat products like sausages and streaky bacon have a relatively high fat content, and if you're a burger fan opt for the varieties made from the leanest meat.

31

Vegetables, salad and fruit

Choose fresh or frozen rather than canned whenever possible and use fresh produce as soon after purchase as you can. The longer fruit and veg are stored before being eaten, the more of their vitamin content is lost. Kale, for example, loses one-third of its vitamin C content within 24 hours of being picked. Commercial freezing is done soon after harvesting so that the vitamin loss is minimised, whereas the high temperatures used in the canning process mean that there may be some vitamin destruction. It's also quite common for sugar to be added, which contributes nothing to the nutritional value.

You really can't have too much from this food group. Apart from all the fibre they give you, eating a lot of vegetables, salad and fruit will boost your levels of important vitamins, especially the so-called 'anti-oxidants'. These are vitamins C and E and beta-carotene which is related to vitamin A, and experts believe they play an important part in protecting you against some forms of cancer and heart disease. Ideally, you should aim for three servings of vegetables or salad and two of fruit each day.

32

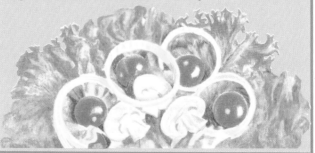

When less is best

While it's not a good idea to go to extremes, there is a case for cutting down on some ingredients of the average diet.

Fats

We all need some fat in our diet to meet our needs for substances called essential fatty acids which help the body maintain itself, However, there is no doubt that most of us get more than the necessary three ounces a day. What's more, the majority of it is likely to be in the form of saturated fats, which mostly come from animal sources.

These are the cause of most concern health-wise, although a study done at Harvard University in the USA reported in 1994 that a type of fat known as trans-fatty acids also appears to increase levels of cholesterol in the blood and make it stickier. This type of fat is found in many margarines and in some prepared foods like biscuits and cakes. They are formed when vegetable oils are chemically treated (hydrogenated) to turn them from liquids to solids.

Know your fats

● **Saturated fats:** foods with a high content include butter, lard and most margarines, hard cheeses such as Cheddar, whole milk, cream and any dairy products not made with skimmed or semi-skimmed milk plus meat such as lamb, pork and beef. They are usually solid at room temperature.

● **Polyunsaturated fats –** such as oils made from vegetables, soya, sunflower, safflower or rapeseed, for example, and butter-substitute spreads which are specifically labelled 'high in poly-unsaturates'.

● **Monounsaturated fats** in practice mean olive oil and this seems to carry considerable bonuses. It is an essential part of the diet of the Greeks, who have one of the lowest rates of heart disease in the world (despite being a nation of smokers!).

33

Blood fats

The fats which circulate in your bloodstream – known as lipids – come in two forms, cholesterol and triglycerides.

High levels of cholesterol are an important risk factor for heart disease. A long-term research project in the USA, known as the Framingham Study, has shown that people with a blood cholesterol level of below 5.0 mmol/litre have a relatively low risk; by contrast, someone with a level of 6.4 mmol/litre or above faces two and a half times the risk of heart disease.

To make the picture still more confusing, cholesterol comes in two forms. The damage is done by the type known as low-density lipoproteins (LDLs) which make the blood clot more easily and are responsible for the deposits known as atheroma which accumulate on your artery walls and impede the blood flow. This process, known as atherosclerosis, can lead to serious health problems such as heart attack and stroke. High-density lipoproteins (HDLs), on the other hand, are thought to be protective against athero-sclerosis.

High levels of triglycerides usually go along with raised cholesterol levels, and are often found in people who are seriously overweight. They are also higher in people who consume a lot of sugar and drink lots of alcohol.

Your body makes a certain amount of lipids for itself, and some foods actually contain cholesterol – notably eggs, liver, kidney and shellfish. However, these are relatively unimportant sources compared with animal fats which appear to increase cholesterol levels and so encourage the development of atherosclerosis. Reducing your overall fat consumption and opting for poly-unsaturated or mono-unsaturated fats will slow or even reverse this process. When it comes to butter or margarine, try to use less of them or opt for low-fat spreads instead, preferably those which are labelled 'high in poly-unsaturates'.

This will have additional benefits. Fats are extremely rich in energy, so eating a lot of them leads to being overweight, in itself a risk factor for heart disease.

The main thing is to try to reduce the total amount of fat in your diet, which means watching out for 'hidden fats' in pastries, pies and salad dressings, for instance. Ultimately, you should aim to have no more than a third of your daily calorie intake in the form of fat.

34

Sugar

The trouble is that, while our bodies – and especially our teeth – would heave a huge sigh of relief if we never touched any kind of sugar again, most of us love the taste. In any form, sugar is pure calories, and contains no nutrients at all, so while it can give you a short-term energy burst, it's not providing anything your body can usefully use. What's more, we often eat it in combination with foods containing high levels of fat – such as chocolate, biscuits and cakes. In the long-term, this is almost bound to put your weight up – see page 51 for guidelines on how heavy you should be. If you really can't face cutting out sugar altogether, try at least to cut down. As far as possible, it's better to educate your palate to get used to less sweetness, but it will also help if you opt for sugar-free alternatives when you can, such as low calorie drinks, fruit canned in juice instead of syrup and look for processed foods such as baked beans which have a reduced sugar content.

Salt

While your body would be content with half a teaspoonful a day, you probably get through five times that. Most of it is already present when you buy your food – makers add it to everything from bread to canned and packet soups and ready-made sauces.

While much research effort has gone into assessing the health effects of a high salt intake, the results are still inconclusive. Studies have demonstrated that a salt-free diet lowers blood pressure dramatically, while those people who only consume a moderate amount are less prone to high blood pressure. Some experts believe that it is the balance between our intake of salt and potassium that counts, and it may be relevant that foods which contain a lot of one tend to be low in the other. Because a high salt intake may be linked to raised blood pressure, which increases the risk of developing heart and kidney disease and strokes, it is worth trying to cut down.

As well as eating fewer packets of crisps, salted nuts and snacks and less bacon and other salted meats, you can help yourself by using less (or none) when cooking and not adding salt to your meals

35

at the table. At the same time, aim to increase the amount of potassium-rich foods you eat – among the richest sources are cabbage, potatoes in their jackets and other fruits including bananas, grapes, grapefruit, melons, oranges and prunes. However, you're likely to be getting enough potassium if you follow the healthy eating guidelines starting on page 27.

Caffeine

Although there is little evidence that it is actually bad for your health, a high daily intake can leave you feeling twitchy and hyped up. Cutting down on coffee and cola or opting for caffeine-free versions is worthwhile, and substitute herbal and fruit teas or mineral water at least some of the time. If nothing else, you'll get a better night's sleep if you keep your caffeine consumption down in the evenings.

Vitamins and minerals

Eating a wide variety of food should ensure that you take in enough of all the different nutrients your body needs. Precisely how much of each you

need is difficult to say – it will depend on all sorts of factors, such as your age, whether you are pregnant, whether you smoke and so on. Most experts believe that it is better to eat well rather than rely on vitamin or mineral supplements. If you get your vitamins A and C from fruit and vegetables, you will also be getting health-promoting fibre – and because they make you feel full, you'll less inclined to eat cakes, biscuits or crisps.

The vitamins in fresh fruit and vegetables are easily destroyed, so try to eat them raw or very lightly cooked as often as possible. Whenever practical, eat them unpeeled and leave preparation until the last minute before you're ready to serve the meal.

Making a move

For many people, the word 'exercise' conjures up a picture of a miserable jogger plodding wearily round streets or parks in all weathers. If that's your view, it's no wonder that you find the prospect of taking more exercise

36

pretty unappealing. In fact, even the miserable jogger would almost certainly say that he felt better for making the effort, but the point is that exercise can and should be enjoyable. If it isn't, you probably won't keep it up for very long, even though you can feel that it's doing you good.

The right kind of exercise can bring all kinds of bonuses – psychological as well as physical. The secret of success, however, is choosing something which you not only enjoy doing, but which is right for you at your particular age and level of fitness, and which will slot relatively easily into your existing lifestyle. It's not a good idea, for example, to start playing squash or to join a high-impact aerobics class once a week as your first step. The physical strain is likely to lead to injuries unless you are already very fit, and you would benefit more from taking less demanding exercise more frequently, at least to begin with.

Whatever you choose to do, you'll find it easier and be less likely to hurt yourself if you always make a point of building 10 minutes' warming up and cooling down into each session. A good teacher will always include these in any kind of class, but the general idea is to get your heart and lungs working and loosen up your muscles and joints with gentle, rhythmic movements similar to those you'll be using when you start exercising for real.

Why bother?

The ideal exercise programme will improve your flexibility and muscular strength

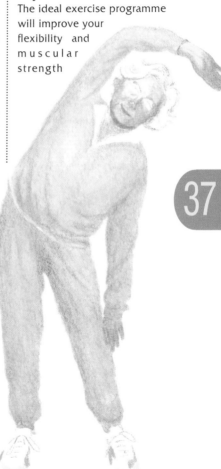

37

and increase your aerobic endurance – in other words, the efficiency of your heart and lungs. Not only will you feel better and fitter, but you can reduce your risk of dying from heart disease. One study of male civil servants done in 1980 found that those who said they exercised regularly had only a third as much heart disease as their more sedentary colleagues. Your heart is a muscle,

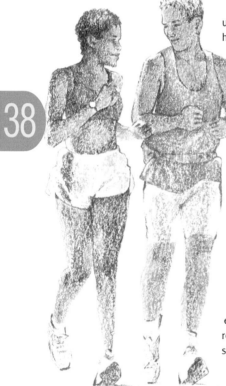

and its job is to pump blood round the body, delivering the oxygen and nutrients to every part, and carrying away waste products. Keeping this vital muscle in peak condition through exercise makes it work more effectively, and means problems are less likely to develop. A healthy heart can pump more blood with each beat, and so beats more slowly, which means it's not having to work so hard.

When you exercise, your body uses up the 'fight or flight' hormones which are released when you're under stress, as well as burning up fats and sugars. There is also some evidence that it improves the balance of lipids in your blood (see page 34) reducing LDLs and tri-glycerides and raising the levels of HDLs.

Toning up your body will mean that your joints, muscles, tendons and ligaments are stronger and more flexible so that you'll be less prone to general aches and pains. What's more, you will be less susceptible to damaging your-self – much back pain, for example, is the result of injuries resulting from quite minor stresses on unfit bodies.

If you opt for something which focuses particularly on one of these areas – say weight training

38

to boost your strength – try and do something else as well which will help with your overall level of fitness.

What's right for you?

Fast walking: good for starters, and all you need is a pair of lightweight, cushioned shoes. Work up from about one mile in 20 minutes, two or three times a week until you can do three miles in about 50 minutes, three times a week. That will be enough to improve your overall fitness, and especially your aerobic endurance so you'll be ready to add more strenuous exercise to your programme if you want to.

Jogging: build up slowly from a mile run – taking as long as you need – twice a week until you can manage two miles in about 20 minutes three times a week. Not only will you notice a big improvement in the efficiency of your heart and lungs, but your legs will be stronger and you may experience the so-called 'runner's

> One study of male civil servants done in 1980 found that those who said they exercised regularly had only a third as much heart disease as their more sedentary colleagues

high'. This is a sensation of well-being which some experts believe results from the release of hormones called endorphins which are the body's natural equivalent of opiate drugs. One word of caution: if you do plan to go jogging, it is sensible to buy the right kind of shoes from a specialist sports shop – trainers and plimsolls don't provide the necessary support and increase your chance of damaging muscles and tendons. When you can't face the weather, 'on-the-spot' jogging on a mini-trampoline indoors may be a more attractive option.

Skipping: can you remember how? It's cheap and convenient – you just need a plastic, rubber or polyurethane rope, a comfortable, even surface and, ideally, a pair of aerobics shoes. Start with just a few minutes a week, gradually increasing the frequency and the time you spend as your fitness improves. It's more tiring than you think, so you may need to rest for a few seconds in each bout at

39

first to get your breath back. As well as improving your aerobic endurance, skipping is good for lower limb muscles, shoulders and back.

Swimming: it's good, all-round exercise and there's little risk of straining muscles or overstressing joints, which makes it a good choice for the seriously unfit. However, you will not see a great deal of benefit if you just cruise slowly up and down the local pool a couple of times a week. Rather, aim to build up your speed and the number of lengths you swim as the weeks pass, including front and back crawl and even butterfly stroke if you can do it. If you're limited to a stately breaststroke, consider joining a class if there are any run locally to learn more strokes and improve your technique. For one thing, it will be less boring than just endless lengths of breaststroke, but equally important, you'll use a wider range of muscles. You may find water aerobics classes on offer at your local pool which can be good fun and make a change from swimming.

Cycling: good for making your heart and lungs work harder and strengthening your legs without putting any stress on your joints. The faster you go and/or the steeper the slope, the harder you have to work. However, bikes don't come cheap, so before you buy one, you do need to be certain you won't go off the idea of cycling regularly (although second-hand ones are much cheaper than new, and bikes don't wear out). It's also worth thinking about local conditions – if there's heavy traffic, you'll not only be breathing in rather a lot of polluted air, you'll also need to be aware of the accident risks. Car and lorry drivers are not always as careful as they should be about the safety of their fellow road-users, and

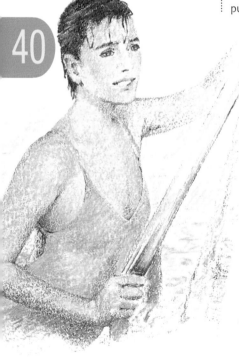

40

Keep exercise boredom at bay

- If possible listen to music or watch television when exercising
- Exercise with other people – remember you should always be able to carry on a conversation when exercising
- Vary the length of your routine,
  e.g. do 20 minutes one day, 30 minutes the next
- Vary the way you are exercising,
  e.g. low effort for 5 minutes, moderate effort for 10 minutes
  low effort for 5 minutes, 10 quick 10 slow, 9 quick 9 slow, etc.
- Combine a number of exercises into your total workout time,
  e.g. warm up for 10 minutes, walk/run for 20 minutes, cycle
  for 20 minutes, and finally stretch and cool off for 10 minutes
  Vary the pattern and length of time for each
- Vary the day on which you exercise
  e.g. don't always cycle 20 minutes on Wednesday

cyclists are very vulnerable, however careful they are themselves when riding. You can, of course, avoid these risks by opting for an exercise bike to use at home. This can be a very accessible way of exercising. It can become repetitive but if you listen to music or watch television and introduce variety into your routine it isn't difficult to stick with it (see the box above).

Rowing: on a machine is a very effective form of exercise, working many different muscle groups and improving muscle weakness. Rowing requires a good technique and it is best to try a rowing machine in a gym under proper supervision and guidance before starting on your own. Rowing on a rowing machine can become repetitive if you let it. See the box 'Keep exercise boredom at bay' for advice.

Dance: we're not talking about throwing yourself around at the occasional party here, but regular sessions of something energetic like rock and roll or salsa are very effective ways of getting fit. Many people have found this is the perfect solution to their motivation problem, because learning to dance properly can be a lot more fun than solo swimming or running, for example. Your options will depend on where you live, but you should be able to find something, either through your local continuing education department or ads in the local paper or Yellow Pages. The popularity of the film 'Strictly

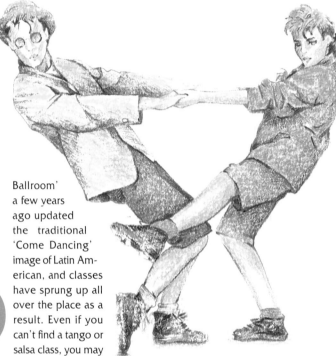

42

Ballroom' a few years ago updated the traditional 'Come Dancing' image of Latin American, and classes have sprung up all over the place as a result. Even if you can't find a tango or salsa class, you may be able to do tap, flamenco or even belly dancing. They're all much more demanding physically than you might think, but classes are usually very sociable and great fun too.

Weight training: the main aim here is to increase your strength and, as you do so, tone up your muscles. Unless you really get interested in weightlifting as a sport or in body-building as an end in itself, you'll need to work out a programme that strengthens and shapes up your muscles

without producing too much bulk. The simplest way is to join a good local gym, where there is a wide range of equipment and qualified instructors to teach you how to use it correctly. Alternatively, you can buy simple equipment, such as a barbell, to use at home, but make sure you have a good instruction book or video to show you the proper way to use it or you could do more harm than good. Regular weight training can improve the shape of your body quite dramatically, but it won't have much effect on your aerobic fitness, so it's a good idea to do some aerobic exercise as well to benefit your heart and lungs. Incidentally, you may well find that your weight goes up as you train, because you're replacing fat with muscle, which is heavier.

Everyday life: as well as building some sort of exercise routine into your life, it's worth trying to develop the habit of being more energetic in general. Simple things, like using stairs instead of lifts, walking to the bus stop beyond your usual one or walking to the shops instead of driving whenever you can, are all worthwhile in fitness terms. The more you do, the easier it is. You'll soon find that heavy jobs in the garden, carrying children or shopping seems to take much less effort than they used to. What's more, if you have to miss out on your usual exercise

routine for a while for some reason, you'll actually be sorry and be keen to get back to it as soon as you can.

One final word of caution: as we've seen earlier in the book, sports injuries are all too common. Many can be avoided with commonsense – having the right shoes, well-maintained equipment, following safety rules and so on – so do take proper care. Should you suffer anything more than a minor injury, it's unwise to ignore it or to go on exercising as this will just make it worse. Rest until you feel all right again, and, if necessary, check out your technique so the same thing doesn't happen again. Equally, you should give yourself a break

43

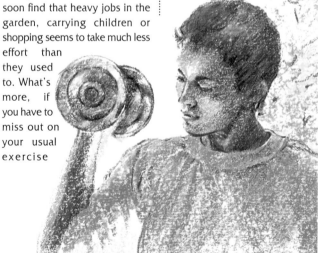

if you feel off-colour or if you have a virus infection such as a cold. There is a slight but real risk that you could damage your heart, so rest until you are back to normal.

Learning to live with stress

Stress seems to be so much part of everyday life in twentieth century Britain that we take it for granted, and blame it for everything from overweight to depression to cancer. Experts disagree about the extent to which being under stress contributes to ill-health and whether it plays a part in causing specific diseases. Nevertheless, there's no doubt that the kind of stress which produces physical or psychological symptoms isn't doing you any good and interferes with your enjoyment of life.

In fact, it's difficult to define exactly what we mean by this everyday word: one person's stress is another's stimulating challenge, and everyone responds differently to pressure and crises. It's easier to pinpoint the signs that you are not coping well with stress, whatever the particular triggers may be in your personal situation.

Signs of stress

- Having trouble getting to sleep, waking up frequently or waking too early in the mornings
- Feeling anxious or on edge for no obvious reason
- Finding it hard to concentrate
- Losing your temper or being irritable with other people
- Becoming indecisive
- Feeling as if your pulse is racing or your heart beating fast or irregularly
- Dry mouth
- 'Butterflies' in your tummy,

44

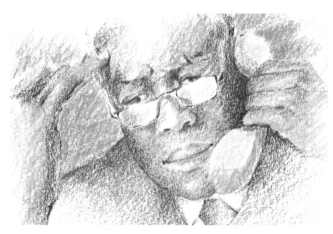

needing to empty your bladder frequently or passing frequent, loose motions.

As you can see, the signs of being under stress are a mixture of physical and psychological sensations, but the origin of them all is in your mental and emotional reactions. It's a myth that it's only the high-powered types leading obviously pressurised lives who suffer from stress-related symptoms. In fact, research suggests that such problems are more common in people who have more ordinary jobs (or no job at all) and who feel that they are not in control of what happens in their lives. Bosses cause more stress than they suffer.

What you can do

There are two main ways of tackling stress:

● Changing those elements in your life which provoke stressful reactions. Unfortunately this isn't always possible – a death in the family, for example, or losing your job are outside your control, and are bound to cause a lot of stress.

● Adapting your response to those things which you can't alter, and learning to accept them or at least cope calmly with them.

> **When you're tense and anxious, the hardest thing to do is relax**

You may be aware that something in your life is putting you under continuous or frequent stress – an unhappy relationship or an awkward boss, for example. Sometimes it is better in the long-run to confront the problem head-on, even if the process is difficult or painful at the time.

Whenever possible, it is worth making a positive attempt to talk over the situation with the person concerned, and see whether the difficulties can't be resolved. In some situations, especially at work, you may need to seek help from someone else – such as the personnel officer or your trade union representative. Similarly, in a personal relationship, outside counselling such as that provided by Relate may be the best way forward.

In any situation where you feel your point of view is being ignored or that you are under pressure to do things you don't want to, you may be able to change things if you learn to be more assertive. This doesn't mean becoming aggressive or losing your temper, but simply making your feelings clear and refusing to be bullied. This isn't always easy to do without help, but many people have benefited from attending

45

assertiveness classes or just from reading one of the widely available books on the subject. Your local library is probably the best place to find out more.

When you're tense and anxious, the hardest thing to do is relax, yet this is what you really need. What's more, relaxing doesn't just mean slumping on the sofa in front of the TV, but rather eliminating all the mental and physical tension which has built up. For some people, an absorbing activity like gardening or a game of badminton may do the trick. For others it's a task unrelated to their everyday concerns, like cooking or listening to music. When relatively simple things like this don't work, it may be worth making an effort to learn specific techniques of relaxation – whether it's deep breathing exercise, meditation or yoga, for example. You'll find plenty of books and videos demonstrating these and related methods of relaxation or alternatively you could look for a local class.

Don't be tempted to soothe your jangled nerves with alcohol. There's no harm in moderate drinking, but alcohol can all too easily become a crutch which you come to rely on when times are difficult. It is a potentially addictive drug and the consequences of becoming dependent on it are far-reaching. As well as changing your personality and making it difficult or impossible to live a normal life, it can damage the liver and have other harmful physical effects. Much better to try and deal with the causes of your stress than masking the symptoms with drink.

If you can train yourself to recognise the symptoms of stress, you can begin to try and change your reactions. Instead of responding furiously when someone cuts you up on the road, or fuming uselessly in a traffic jam, for example, you'll make a conscious decision to accept the inevitable calmly. Try to remember that getting all wound up doesn't change the situation one iota, it just makes it harder to deal with.

46

Smoking

Having read this far, you can be under no illusions about the effect of smoking on your health. Since the first report of a study by Sir Richard Doll in 1950 which proved the link between lung cancer and smoking, the evidence that smoking damages your health has continued to accumulate. In 1991, a study of 40,000 doctors, begun in 1951 by Sir Richard Doll, showed that the death rates in those who smoked were three times higher than those in non-smokers. Studies in the USA looking at the death rates of middle-aged men between 1984 and 1988 showed that three times as many smokers died as non-smokers.

There is some good news, however. Give up and your risk of dying prematurely as a result of smoking starts dropping straightaway. Provided you haven't already developed lung cancer or serious heart or lung disease, you will avoid most of the smoking-related risk.

● Twenty-four hours after you smoked your last cigarette, your body will have got rid of the carbon monoxide

> **Give up and your risk of dying prematurely as a result of smoking starts dropping straightaway**

● After two or three days, the clotting factors in your blood can be back to normal, reducing the risk of thrombosis

● By the end of a year, your risk of having a heart attack will have dropped by around half

● After five to ten years, your risk of smoking-related illness is virtually the same as that of someone who's never smoked

● In the last 15 years, around 1,000 people a day have given up – if they can do it, so can you.

Lots of people don't manage to give up the first time they try, but this doesn't mean they can never succeed. You can still try again, and remember that there are plenty of people only too willing to help. Ring Quitline for advice and support, useful booklets, and details of a non-smoking support group near you (0171 487 3000, office hours 7 days a week).

Six steps to success

The first, and certainly the most important, step is to make up your mind that you WANT to stop. This is harder than it sounds, and can take time, but it really is the key to success. This doesn't mean putting off the decision indefinitely, but it does mean thinking about why you want to do it and preparing yourself psychologically.

Remember that the withdrawal symptoms are NOT unbearable, and normally disappear within three weeks anyway. If you're worried about how you'll cope, ask your doctor about nicotine replacements – such as patches and gum – and other aids which you can buy over the counter at the chemist.

Analyse your smoking habits so you'll be prepared for the most difficult times – say after a meal, making a phone call or after making love. Plan to have alternatives available – a glass of orange juice, some chewing gum or whatever.

Think one day at a time – that way you'll avoid wondering how you'll cope without smoking for the rest of your life. Don't forget that you were once a non-smoker, however long ago, and you didn't miss it then!

Ignore anyone who tells you that just one cigarette won't hurt – it will. Before you know it, you could be back to 20 a day!

Concentrate on what you're gaining, not on what you're giving up. For some people the most important thing is freedom from addiction, for others it's the money they're saving.

48

Check out your health

Medical science can already treat and even cure many conditions that would have been fatal just a generation ago, and the list is growing longer all the time. In virtually all cases, however, the odds on recovery are very much better if the condition is spotted as early as possible, so that the necessary treatment can be given straightaway. This is why screening programmes have been introduced to pick up the first signs of a potentially serious problem – such as changes in the cervix which could eventually develop into cancer. Some forms of screening are offered to everyone, others will only be needed by people who are thought to be at risk from a particular illness, perhaps because it runs in their families. Doctors are also on the look-out for other factors which could make you more prone to illness later in life, even though you may be fine at the moment. For example, raised blood pressure and obesity come into this category because they may eventually cause trouble if not tackled now.

As well as the checks which should be done by doctors and other qualified people, there are some which you should carry out yourself at regular intervals so as to be aware of any changes which may need medical attention. Women should learn 'breast awareness', for instance, while men should check their testes, and both should keep an eye on any moles or marks on their skin and tell their GP about any visible changes.

> **The odds on recovery are very much better if the condition is spotted as early as possible**

49

Your test card
Blood pressure

Everyone should have this checked at their GP's surgery every five years (unless it is raised, when it will be checked more frequently), because it can rise without you having any symptoms. Raised blood pressure (hypertension) is associated with an increased risk of heart disease and other circulation problems such as strokes. Depending on the level of your blood pressure, your GP may prescribe tablets to lower it, and anyone who smokes will be very strongly advised to stop. In addition, the doctor may recommend that you lose weight if necessary, take exercise and do whatever you can to minimise stress.

Blood tests

These will normally only be done if your doctor thinks there is a particular reason why you need them. For example, a woman of child-bearing age may need to be checked for immunity to rubella (or German measles). Although this is a very minor illness in itself, catching it in early pregnancy can harm the unborn baby, and anyone who is not already immune should be immunised before planning to conceive.

Similarly, if your doctor thinks you are at high risk of developing heart disease, perhaps because of a family history and the presence of other risk factors such as smoking and high blood pressure, he or she may want to check your cholesterol levels.

Sometimes blood tests may help in the diagnosis of specific illnesses, but they are not normally needed as part of a routine check-up.

50

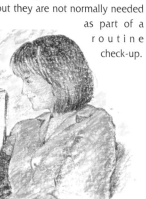

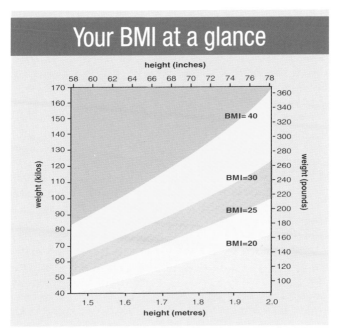

Your BMI at a glance

Weight

Your doctor will be concerned if you are far heavier than you should be for your height and build, but also if you are definitely under-weight. He or she may check your correct weight on a height/weight chart, or use the so-called BMI (or body mass index). This is calculated by dividing your weight in kilos by your height in metres squared. The recommended range is from 20 to 25, the blue shaded area in our diagram.

Although experts are beginning to take a more relaxed view about mild overweight, a BMI outside the acceptable range, or carrying more than half a stone (3 kg) of surplus fat still means you need to do something about shedding the extra weight. People who weigh too much are putting extra strain on their bodies, especially their hearts, and are also more prone to develop health problems such as high blood pressure, non insulin-dependent diabetes and osteoarthritis. Early in 1995, one report suggested that slightly overweight people actually live longer than their really skinny counterparts, but there were probably other factors involved, and the evidence is not strong enough to justify complacency.

51

You should aim to shift the excess pounds slowly and steadily by eating a well-balanced diet, cutting right down on all foods that are high in fat and/or sugar. Your GP will be able to give you a diet sheet if you need more specific guidelines, or may have a dietitian working with him to whom he can refer you for advice.

Whatever you do, steer clear of crash diets. For one thing, you'll put all the weight back on once you return to normal eating. For another, you may be depriving your body of vital nutrients which it needs to maintain good health. There is evidence that 'yo-yo' dieting – losing then regaining weight repeatedly – is actually unhealthy in itself. Keeping off the weight you've lost means changing your eating habits for good, and if you follow the guidelines for healthy eating on pages 27–36, your weight should remain pretty stable.

Although we are most aware of the increased health risks posed by excess weight, being under-weight isn't good for you either. Your life expectancy will be greatest if you can keep yourself within the average weight range for your height and build. Recent research

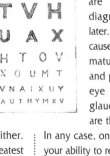

also suggests that the way your weight is distributed around your body may also have a bearing on your susceptibility to some illnesses. In general, it seems that you'll be healthier if your excess weight is spread round evenly, or with most of it around your hips and thighs than if you have a 'spare tyre' round your middle or a pot belly. In other words, it's better to be the traditional British 'pear shape' than apple-shaped!

Vision

Since charges were introduced for sight tests, the number of people having them has dropped. This might not seem to matter much when you are sure you can see as well as ever, but one consequence is that some conditions which used to be spotted early on during examination of the eyes are now not being diagnosed until much later. Changes in the eye caused by non-insulin (or mature onset) diabetes and potentially serious eye problems such as glaucoma and cataract are the main examples. In any case, once you're over 40, your ability to read without glasses may well start to deteriorate, so it's worth getting your eyes checked regularly as a precaution. Your vision

52

may have got worse so slowly that you haven't noticed, but once you get new glasses, you'll realise just how much you've been missing!

Cervical smear

All women between the ages of 20 and 64 should automatically be invited to come to their GP's surgery for a smear test at least once every five years. The test involves gently scraping a few cells from the cervix which are then sent off to a lab for analysis. The aim is to detect any changes which might one day develop into cancer if neglected. Most people will get the all clear within a couple of weeks, but occasionally you might to asked to go back for a repeat test. This is often because the first one didn't produce a satisfactory result, but there's no need to worry even if abnormal cells are found because treatment is simple and normally very effective.

Mammography

All women aged between 50 and 64 will be automatically sent an invitation once every three years to go to their nearest breast screening centre for a mammogram. This is a specialised kind of X-ray which picks up abnormalities in the breast tissue, which may sometimes be the early stages of breast cancer. In fact, only a small minority of women who need further investigations as a result of a mammogram are found

to have cancer; 90 per cent of all lumps turn out to be benign and easily dealt with. Even when the diagnosis is one of cancer, early treatment is often successful. It's natural to be nervous about the prospect of having this test, and hard not to be worried if it shows up something that needs further investigation. Nevertheless, it really is worth plucking up your courage to keep the appointment, so that if there is anything wrong, it can be spotted and the necessary treatment given as soon as possible.

DIY checks
Breast awareness

Even before you're old enough to be offered mammography, it's a good idea to train yourself to check for any changes in your breasts. The best way to approach this is to get into the habit of looking carefully at both breasts in a full-length mirror, preferably at the same point each month in your menstrual cycle. Be alert for any changes in shape or size, any puckering of the skin and any changes in texture such as small lumps. If you want to do more, ask your GP to show you how to feel your breasts for any lumps – it's quite easy to do, but not strictly necessary provided you keep on the look-out for any visible changes. If you do notice anything, tell your doctor as soon as possible. The strong likelihood is

53

that it will be nothing to worry about, but it's best to make sure.

Testicle awareness

These days testicular cancer is no longer the major killer of young men that it used to be. Most patients with the condition are cured, even if it is detected at a late stage.

Although lumps are very common, fortunately the vast majority are not cancerous. However, whether out of fear or ignorance many men do not seem to notice any changes in their testicles, or to ignore them if they do notice. To allay anxiety, and to avoid the need for major surgery and chemotherapy, early diagnosis is very desirable. The best way to do this is to develop the habit of examining yourself about once a month, preferably after a shower or bath when the scrotum is relaxed. First note the size and weight of each testicle – it doesn't matter if they're different sizes but they should weigh about the same. Then use your fingers and thumbs to feel for any lumps, swellings or unevenness. You will probably be able to feel the fine tube which carries sperm at the back and top of each testicle, but otherwise the texture should be smooth. If you do notice any changes, tell your doctor as soon as possible. Chances are it will be nothing serious, but if it should turn out to be cancer, the more quickly it is found and treated, the better.

You pay your money...

Private health insurance schemes offer you the opportunity to have a complete health screen and anyone can go provided they can pay the necessary fee. Most organisations offer a range of options, from a complete overhaul to specialised screening for a man or a woman. Both sexes can have heart and lung tests, blood pressure checks, blood analysis and urine checks and BMI measurement. Opting for a 'well woman screening' means you'll get a more limited range of checks, but it will include breast checks (and a mammogram if you're over 50), plus a smear test and pelvic examination. Having a private mammogram means you can choose to be screened more frequently – say every two years (as in most European countries) rather than every three as under the NHS scheme. This obviously means that an early cancer may be picked up more quickly and so have an even better chance of successful treatment.

In fact, most of these tests should be available through the NHS, although some will only be done if there is a reason why you need them. In any case, if you do choose a private check, the results will be sent to your GP within a couple of weeks, and you'll be able to discuss the results with him or her.

Paper tigers

You could be forgiven for thinking that all this effort to improve your health would be wasted because the environment in which you live is so hazardous anyway. Almost every day there are scare stories in the media about some newly discovered danger with serious implications for the health of the nation. The risks apparently range from radiation to petrol by-products, from fertilisers to pollution and from food additives to insecticides. The one thing they all have in common is that there is supposedly little or nothing we can do to protect ourselves from potential harm. Blaming big business is easier than modifying our own un-healthy life-styles.

While there may often be a kernel of truth in such stories, it is important to get the risks into pers-pective. Even if we assume that some people may die as a result of encountering this type of hazard, the risk for any one individual is minuscule compared to the risk of dying as a result of smoking or crossing a busy road, for example. It's also necessary to think about the balance between benefits and risks in some instances – such as insecticides, fertilisers and food additives. Whatever else, people in all countries are now living longer than their parents or grandparents.

Radiation

In the past, most worries were related to the possible dangers from nuclear power generation, but more recently natural forms such as radon gas and ultraviolet radiation from the sun have been cropping up in the headlines as well. Although local residents are still con-cerned about the apparent 'cancer clus-ters' in areas close to nuclear installations, especially Sellafield, repeated scientific investigations

55

have not so far established any incontrovertible evidence of a link. Countries such as France and Sweden rely on nuclear power for much of their electricity – half the total in Sweden.

A greater, although still relatively minor, risk is faced by those living in areas where a naturally radioactive gas called radon is present in high concentrations. This is a particular problem in parts of Cornwall, for example, but people living in affected areas can apply to have their homes modified to improve ventilation and so reduce the level of radon. For people in other parts of the country, radon is simply part of the natural background radiation which is (and has always been) ever-present and unchangeable, and in any case appears to present no real threat to health.

Reports about the reduction in the ozone layer of the atmosphere which protects us from solar radiation undoubtedly worry many people. Scientifically, the jury is still out on the seriousness and possible implications of such changes, but one positive consequence is increasing awareness of the dangers of skin cancer resulting from too much sunshine. Sunbathing (and especially sunburn) are undoubtedly bad for your skin, so covering up and using plenty of the right type of sunscreen are sensible precautions for everyone (see page 19).

Pollution

While atmospheric pollution caused by smoking chimneys may have almost disappeared, it has been replaced by the by-products of the internal combustion engine. This has coincided with a rise in the numbers of people suffering from allergic conditions such as asthma and hayfever and in cases of bronchitis and other chest problems. While most doctors agree that the two facts are connected, it seems likely that pollution isn't causing the illnesses directly, but rather setting off attacks in those people who are already susceptible. Whatever the truth, there is little the individual can do to change things until or unless governments and drivers agree on some way to cut down the use of motor transport of all kinds – or at least pay the cost of

56

reducing the amount of pollutants they produce.

Poisons in petrol

The last 10 years have seen moves towards reducing the amounts of lead released into the atmosphere by petrol-powered vehicles. Lead is poisonous even in low concentrations and has an adverse effect on health, especially on children living close to major roads. More drivers are now choosing lead-free petrol, and new cars are fitted with catalytic converters to cut down on the amount of noxious substances escaping from their exhausts. The MOT test now incorporates checks on exhaust gases which mean older cars may need minor modifications to reduce the toxicity of their exhaust fumes as far as possible. No doubt all this is helpful to some degree, but anxiety is now being focused on the benzene in lead-free petrol. The real problem is traffic density, and progress on finding a solution is unlikely to be rapid until drivers are persuaded to make less use of their vehicles. Meanwhile, although there is no doubt that lead and other exhaust pollutants do us no good, few people will experience any serious ill-effects and there is little any one of us can do to change the situation overnight.

Food additives

Additives with E numbers got a really bad name back in the eighties when they were suspected of causing all manner of illnesses. In fact, the dangers were wildly exaggerated and often based on misunderstandings. For one thing, many of the substances given E numbers as part of an agreed international labelling system are perfectly 'natural' chemicals and found in plants, fruits or other ordinary foods. Some additives were alleged to be carcinogenic (cancer-causing) following experiments with animals, even though there was no evidence that they would have the same effect on humans, and despite the fact that many of the poor animals only developed

57

tumours when fed the offending substances in enormous doses. The opposition to additives often ignored the fact that many of them were preservatives, making food safer to eat, and certainly carrying fewer risks to health than alternative ways of conserving food such as smoking, salting and pickling.

Regulations about testing and which additives may be used and in what quantities are stringent, and there is very little chance that you could do yourself harm by consuming food or drinks containing them. There are some good reasons for reducing the proportion of processed food in your overall diet, but avoiding additives comes pretty low on the list.

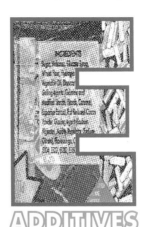

ADDITIVES

Agricultural chemicals

The widespread use of fertilisers, pesticides and animal feed additives has revolutionised farming, bringing bigger crops with fewer obvious blemishes. Moulds and fungi growing on vegetables and nuts have been linked with some types of cancer. Chemicals reduce these risks. The downside is that we have little or no idea what residues we may be consuming, and what effects if any they might have on our health.

Despite occasional scares like the one concerning allegedly contaminated apple juice in 1984, there is no hard evidence of any substantial harm to consumers resulting from the use of such chemicals. People who prefer to err on the side of caution can opt for organically grown fruit, veg and other products (if they are willing to pay the premium producers' charge to cover their extra costs) and drink only bottled water for example. A less extreme line is to make sure you always wash all fruit, veg and salad before eating them to get rid of any chemical residues lingering on the surfaces. Most of us, however, will simply go on eating the foods we enjoy without worrying too much and are likely to suffer no ill-effects to our health as a consequence.

Your personal action plan

I f, after reading all this, you are inspired to make changes to your lifestyle for the sake of good health, where should you start? The answer depends to a great extent on the way you live now. Your personality will also be a factor – you'll do better if you tailor your transformation to suit your personal make-up.

A plodder or a plunger?

● Plodders like to go about things calmly and in an organised way, taking one step at a time. Think about the areas in your life where change is most urgent, then break them down into manageable chunks. You may like to set yourself weekly goals – say at the end of seven days you will have switched to low-calorie drinks and spreads and swapped from whole to semi-skimmed milk, for example. Making a list of your aims helps you to see where you're heading, and you can give yourself the satisfaction of ticking off each item once you've achieved it.

● Plungers can't bear half measures. As far as you're concerned, it's all or nothing. This may well work, provided you don't aim to change every aspect of your life all at once. You

59

BRITISH MEDICAL ASSOCIATION

might do better to concentrate on one aspect at a time – say devising an exercise plan and really getting into that before you start revising your diet. This doesn't mean it will take for ever, but it will be less to cope with all in one go, and should be more achievable.

Sort out your priorities

Whichever approach you take, it's worth thinking about your priorities before you start. Ask yourself where you personally are in greatest need of improvement. Most of us can pick one aspect where we know we are weakest, so why not start with that? Once you've got over your biggest hurdle, the others will seem far less daunting, because you'll have proved that you can change if you want to.

Planning a healthier future

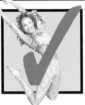

Your diet isn't too far off the ideal, and you don't drink or smoke, but you are a confirmed couch potato who never walks when you can drive. In this case, a fitness programme should be your top priority, and you can get round to changing your eating habits later. ☐

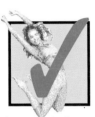

Smokers can't be in any doubt about their first priority: give up! Apart from the obvious damage you know it's doing to your lungs, it is also bad for your heart and circulation and makes you more susceptible to a number of other diseases, including some forms of cancer. Make up your mind to do it, then get help if you need it. There are plenty of aids to willpower around (see page 48) and your GP will be keen to advise and encourage you. ☐

60

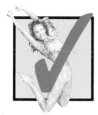

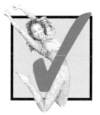

When you know that you have a weight problem and eat too much of the wrong foods, make this your starting point. As we've seen, diet is thought to play a role in the development of certain cancers, and being seriously overweight can be a risk factor in heart disease as well as possibly contributing to the onset of one kind of diabetes. Excess weight also puts extra strain on the joints, creating problems for anyone with arthritis. Add to this the beneficial effects of a diet that is high in fibre, fruit and veg and low on sugar and fat, and it's obvious that moving towards the kind of healthy eating plan outlines on pages 27–36 will bring enormous benefits. You'll know by now whether you need to make minor or major adjustments to the way you eat, and even a gradual approach is worth starting as soon as possible. Once you've taken the first steps, other changes can be introduced over the coming weeks and months. ☐

Drinking isn't unhealthy in moderation, but making an effort to keep your alcohol consumption inside reasonable limits (see page 15) is certainly worthwhile. This can be difficult if your social life revolves around the pub or wine bar or if social drinking goes with your job, but when you do try to cut down you'll almost certainly find you are not alone. If you find the task just too difficult to handle without help, you might like to contact an organisation like Drinkwise (0171 413 1888) who will know how you feel and offer advice and support. ☐

Stick with it!

It's important that you don't think of all these changes as the equivalent of going on a slimming diet – three months of torture and it'll all be over. What you're aiming at are changes that will become a permanent way of life and seem so natural that you don't even think of going back to your old lifestyle.

61

FAMILY DOCTOR PUBLICATIONS

63